20 SMOOTHIES FOR KIDNEY HEALTH

A tasty strategy for preventing and treating kidney issues

By

Donald V. Schaper

DISCLAIMER

TABLE OF CONTENT

Conclusion

INTRODUCTION

Kidney health is an important aspect of overall wellness, as the kidneys play a crucial role in removing waste and excess fluids from the body. Unfortunately, kidney issues are becoming increasingly common, affecting millions of people worldwide. Fortunately, there are many ways to prevent and treat kidney issues, including diet and nutrition.

Smoothies have gained popularity in recent years as a delicious and nutritious way to incorporate fruits, vegetables, and other healthy ingredients into our daily diets. They can be a particularly useful tool for those looking to improve their kidney health, as they can provide a variety of vitamins, minerals, and antioxidants that support healthy kidney function.

In this article, we will explore the benefits of smoothies for kidney health and how they can be used as a tasty strategy for preventing and treating kidney issues. We will discuss some of the best ingredients to include in kidney-friendly smoothies, as well as tips for creating delicious and nutritious blends. So, whether you are looking to support your kidney health or simply enjoy a tasty and healthy beverage, read on to discover the benefits of smoothies for kidney health.

Smoothies are a convenient and easy way to consume a variety of fruits and vegetables in one delicious drink. This is particularly beneficial for those with kidney issues, as a healthy diet is essential for maintaining kidney health. A diet that is high in fruits and vegetables has been shown to reduce the risk of chronic kidney disease, and may also help to manage symptoms in those with existing kidney issues.

Smoothies can also be customized to meet individual nutritional needs. For example, those with kidney issues may need to limit their intake of certain minerals, such as potassium and phosphorus, which can build up in the body and cause further damage to the kidneys. By carefully selecting the ingredients in their smoothies, individuals can tailor their beverages to their unique nutritional needs and support healthy kidney function.

In addition to providing essential vitamins and minerals, smoothies can also help to keep the body hydrated. Proper hydration is essential for kidney health, as it helps to flush out toxins and waste products from the body. Smoothies can be made with a variety of hydrating ingredients, such as coconut water, cucumber, and watermelon, to support optimal hydration levels.

Smoothies are a delicious and nutritious way to support kidney health. By incorporating a variety of fruits and vegetables into their daily diets, individuals can support healthy kidney function and prevent or manage kidney issues. With a bit of creativity and experimentation, anyone can create delicious and kidney-friendly smoothies that support their overall health and well-being.

CHAPTER ONE

Kidneys-The Body's Workhorses

The kidneys are two bean-shaped organs located in the lower back, one on either side of the spine. They are responsible for filtering waste products and excess fluid from the blood, which are then excreted in the form of urine. Additionally, the kidneys play a crucial role in maintaining proper fluid balance, regulating blood pressure, and producing hormones that help to regulate red blood cell production and bone health.

The kidneys are often referred to as the body's workhorses, as they work tirelessly to perform these vital functions. They are responsible for filtering approximately 120-150 quarts of blood per day, removing waste products and excess fluid, and returning essential nutrients and water to the bloodstream. The kidneys also play a crucial role in regulating electrolyte levels in the body, including sodium, potassium, and calcium, which are necessary for proper muscle and nerve function.

The kidneys are vital organs in the human body responsible for several important functions. They are located on either side of the spine, just below the ribcage, and are responsible for filtering the blood and removing waste products from the body.

One of the primary functions of the kidneys is to regulate the body's fluid balance. They do this by filtering the blood and removing excess water, salts, and other substances that the body does not need. This helps to maintain proper hydration levels and prevent fluid buildup in the body.

Another important function of the kidneys is to regulate the body's electrolyte balance. Electrolytes are minerals such as sodium, potassium, and calcium that are essential for many bodily functions. The kidneys help to maintain proper levels of electrolytes in the blood by either reabsorbing them or excreting them in the urine.

The kidneys also play a crucial role in regulating blood pressure. They do this by producing a hormone called renin, which helps to regulate blood volume and maintain blood pressure within a healthy range.

In addition to these functions, the kidneys also help to remove waste products from the body, such as urea and creatinine. They do this by filtering the blood and excreting these waste products in the urine.

The kidneys are incredibly important organs that play a crucial role in maintaining proper bodily function. By regulating fluid and electrolyte balance, blood pressure, and removing waste products from the body, the kidneys help to keep us healthy and functioning at our best.

Many factors can contribute to the development of kidney issues, including high blood pressure, diabetes, and a family history of kidney disease. Lifestyle factors, such as smoking and a poor diet, can also increase the risk of kidney issues.

Fortunately, there are many things that individuals can do to support healthy kidney function and prevent or manage kidney issues. This includes maintaining a healthy diet that is rich in fruits and vegetables, staying hydrated, exercising regularly, and avoiding smoking and excessive alcohol consumption.

Smoothies can be a convenient and delicious way to support healthy kidney function as part of a healthy diet. By incorporating a variety of fruits and vegetables into their smoothies, individuals can provide their bodies with the nutrients and hydration necessary to support optimal kidney function. Additionally, by carefully selecting ingredients that are low in potassium and phosphorus, individuals with kidney issues can customize their smoothies to meet their unique nutritional needs and support kidney health.

Incorporating smoothies into a kidney-healthy diet can be a helpful strategy for individuals who are looking to manage or prevent kidney issues. Smoothies can be an easy and convenient way to consume a wide range of nutrients, including vitamins, minerals, and antioxidants, which are essential for maintaining optimal health.

Some of the best ingredients to include in kidney-healthy smoothies include low-potassium fruits such as berries, apples, and grapes, as well as leafy green vegetables like spinach and kale, which are rich in antioxidants and other nutrients that support kidney health.

Additionally, low-fat dairy products such as Greek yogurt and skim milk can provide a good source of protein without overloading the body with excess potassium.

When making smoothies for kidney health, it is important to avoid high-potassium ingredients such as bananas, oranges, and avocados, as well as high-phosphorus ingredients such as chocolate and nuts. Individuals with kidney issues should also be careful not to over-consume protein, as excess protein can put additional strain on the kidneys.

Smoothies can be a delicious and versatile way to support kidney health, and there are many recipes and combinations to choose from. With a little creativity and careful ingredient selection, individuals can enjoy a wide range of tasty and nutritious smoothies that support optimal kidney function and overall health.

CHAPTER TWO

THE DIETARY BASIS OF KIDNEY DISEASE

The kidneys play a vital role in filtering waste products from the blood and excreting them in the urine. However, when the kidneys are damaged or diseased, they may not be able to perform this function effectively. This can lead to the buildup of waste products and other harmful substances in the body, which can cause a range of health problems.

One of the primary causes of kidney disease is poor diet. A diet that is high in salt, sugar, and unhealthy fats can put a strain on the kidneys and increase the risk of developing kidney disease. Additionally, a diet that is low in nutrients, such as fruits and vegetables, can also increase the risk of kidney disease.

One of the key dietary factors that can contribute to kidney disease is a high intake of salt. When the body consumes too much salt, the kidneys must work harder to remove it from the blood. This can lead to damage and inflammation in the kidneys over time. High salt intake can also lead to high blood pressure, which is a major risk factor for kidney disease.

Another dietary factor that can contribute to kidney disease is a high intake of sugar. When the body consumes too much sugar, it can lead to insulin resistance and inflammation, which can damage the kidneys. Additionally, high sugar intake can lead to obesity and type 2 diabetes, both of which are major risk factors for kidney disease.

A diet that is low in nutrients, such as fruits and vegetables, can also increase the risk of kidney disease. Fruits and vegetables are rich in antioxidants, vitamins, and minerals that are important for kidney health. When the body does not receive enough of these nutrients, it can lead to inflammation and damage in the kidneys.

The dietary basis of kidney disease is largely influenced by a diet that is high in salt, sugar, and unhealthy fats, and low in nutrients such as fruits and vegetables. By making healthy dietary choices, individuals can help to prevent and manage kidney disease and maintain optimal kidney health.

Kidney disease can be caused by various factors, including genetic predisposition, infections, medications, and most commonly, an unhealthy diet. Consuming a diet high in sodium, saturated and trans fats, processed foods, and added sugars, and low in fiber, fruits, and vegetables can put a strain on the kidneys and increase the risk of developing kidney disease.

Sodium, for example, is a major component of table salt, which is commonly added to processed foods and fast foods. Consuming high levels of sodium can lead to high blood pressure, which can damage the kidneys and cause kidney disease. Additionally, a diet high in saturated and trans fats can increase the risk of developing high cholesterol and cardiovascular disease, which can also damage the kidneys.

On the other hand, consuming a diet rich in plant-based foods, such as fruits, vegetables, legumes, nuts, and seeds, can support kidney health. These foods are rich in vitamins, minerals, fiber, and antioxidants that can reduce inflammation and oxidative stress in the body, which can contribute to kidney disease. Additionally, plant-based foods are generally low in sodium and saturated fats, making them a healthier option for the kidneys.

It is also important to note that adequate hydration is crucial for kidney health. Drinking enough water helps to flush out waste and toxins from the body, reducing the strain on the kidneys. Not drinking enough water can lead to dehydration and a buildup of waste products, which can contribute to kidney disease.

Maintaining a healthy diet that is low in sodium, saturated, and trans fats, and added sugars, and high in plant-based foods and water can support kidney health and prevent the development of kidney disease.

In addition to a healthy diet, other lifestyle factors can support kidney health and prevent kidney disease. Regular exercise, for example, can help to reduce the risk of developing high blood pressure, obesity, and diabetes, all of which are risk factors for kidney disease.

Avoiding smoking and excessive alcohol consumption can also support kidney health. Smoking can damage blood vessels and reduce blood flow to the kidneys, while excessive alcohol consumption can lead to high blood pressure and dehydration, both of which can contribute to kidney disease.

Regular check-ups with a healthcare provider can also help to identify any potential kidney issues early on and prevent them from progressing to more serious conditions. Tests such as urine and blood tests can detect changes in kidney function, allowing for early intervention and treatment.

Incorporating smoothies into one's diet can also be a delicious and convenient way to support kidney health. Smoothies made with kidney-friendly ingredients such as leafy greens, berries, citrus fruits, and low-sugar plant milk can provide essential nutrients while also promoting hydration.

CHAPTER THREE

KIDNEY FRIENDLY FOODS

The kidneys are vital organs that perform several functions in the body, including filtering waste and excess fluids from the blood, regulating electrolyte balance, and producing hormones that help control blood pressure and red blood cell production. A healthy diet plays a crucial role in maintaining optimal kidney function and preventing kidney disease. Eating kidney-friendly foods can help reduce the workload on the kidneys and prevent complications associated with kidney disease. In this article, we will explore some kidney-friendly foods that can help promote healthy kidney function and prevent kidney disease.

A kidney-friendly diet is an important aspect of managing kidney disease and preventing further damage to the kidneys. Here are some examples of kidney-friendly foods:

- Berries: Berries are rich in antioxidants, which can help to reduce inflammation and protect against cellular damage. Blueberries, raspberries, strawberries, and blackberries are all excellent choices.

- Leafy greens: Leafy greens such as spinach, kale, and collard greens are rich in vitamins and minerals, and low in potassium and phosphorus, making them ideal for people with kidney disease.

- Citrus fruits: Citrus fruits such as oranges, lemons, and limes are high in vitamin C, which can help to protect against cellular damage and inflammation. They are also low in potassium and a good source of hydration.

- Low-sugar plant milk: Plant-based milk such as almond milk, cashew milk, and coconut milk can be a good source of protein and calcium, and are generally lower in phosphorus than dairy milk.

- Low-potassium fruits: Fruits such as apples, grapes, and peaches are low in potassium, making them a good choice for people with kidney disease who need to limit their potassium intake.

- Whole grains: Whole grains such as brown rice, quinoa, and whole wheat pasta can be a good source of fiber and nutrients, while also being lower in phosphorus than refined grains.

- Fish: Certain types of fish, such as salmon and tuna, are rich in omega-3 fatty acids, which can help to reduce inflammation and protect against heart disease. They are also a good source of high-quality protein.

- Cauliflower: A great source of vitamin C and fiber, and low in potassium, cauliflower can be roasted, mashed, or added to soups and stews.

- Blueberries: High in antioxidants and low in potassium, blueberries are a great addition to smoothies or oatmeal.

- Garlic: Helps to lower cholesterol levels and blood pressure, garlic can be added to a variety of dishes for flavor.

- Red bell peppers: A good source of vitamin C and low in potassium, red bell peppers can be roasted or eaten raw in salads.

- Onions: Low in potassium and high in flavor, onions can be added to a variety of dishes for flavor.

- Apples: High in fiber and vitamin C, apples make a great snack or can be added to smoothies or salads.

- Cabbage: Low in potassium and high in vitamin C and fiber, cabbage can be roasted or added to soups and stews.

- Radishes: Low in potassium and high in vitamin C, radishes can be eaten raw or roasted.

- Pineapple: Contains an enzyme called bromelain, which helps to reduce inflammation, pineapple can be added to smoothies or eaten on its own.

It is important to remember that everyone's nutritional needs are different, and consulting with a healthcare professional or registered dietitian can help determine the best kidney-friendly diet plan for an individual's specific needs.

CHAPTER FOUR

KIDNEY ENEMY FOODS

In contrast to kidney-friendly foods, some types of food can harm the kidneys and make them work harder than they should. These foods are commonly referred to as "kidney enemy foods." Consuming too much of these foods can lead to the development of kidney disease or exacerbate existing kidney problems.

Kidney-enemy foods are foods that can cause damage or worsen the health of the kidneys. These foods are high in sodium, potassium, and phosphorus, which are minerals that the kidneys need to filter from the blood. When there is an excess of these minerals, the kidneys have to work harder to remove them, leading to strain and damage to the organ.

Some of the most common kidney enemy foods include processed foods, fast food, canned and packaged foods, salty snacks, and sugary drinks. These foods are often high in sodium, which can raise blood pressure and increase the risk of kidney damage.

Additionally, high-potassium foods like bananas, oranges, tomatoes, and spinach can also be harmful to the kidneys, especially for those with kidney disease or reduced kidney function. Phosphorus-rich foods like cheese, nuts, and whole grains can also contribute to kidney damage over time.

Individuals with kidney issues need to be aware of these kidney-enemy foods and limit their intake as much as possible. Instead, opting for kidney-friendly foods like fresh fruits and vegetables, lean proteins, and whole grains can help to support kidney health and function.

Here are some examples of kidney enemy foods:

- Processed foods: Packaged, processed foods are often high in sodium, which can be harmful to the kidneys. Excess sodium can cause the body to retain water and increase blood pressure, which puts added strain on the kidneys.

- Red meat: Red meat is high in protein and phosphorus, which can be difficult for the kidneys to process. Consuming too much red meat can increase the risk of kidney disease and may worsen existing kidney problems.

- Sugary drinks: Sugary drinks like soda and fruit juice are high in sugar and calories, which can lead to weight gain and high blood sugar levels. High blood sugar levels can damage the kidneys over time, increasing the risk of kidney disease.

- Alcohol: Excessive alcohol consumption can lead to dehydration and put extra strain on the kidneys. Over time, heavy drinking can lead to kidney damage and may increase the risk of kidney disease.

- Salt: Consuming too much salt can increase blood pressure and lead to kidney damage. It is recommended to limit daily sodium intake to less than 2,300 mg per day.

- Caffeine: Caffeine can increase blood pressure and cause dehydration, which can be harmful to the kidneys. It is recommended to limit daily caffeine intake to less than 400 mg per day.

It is important to note that moderation is key when it comes to these kidney-enemy foods. Occasional consumption is unlikely to cause harm, but regular or excessive consumption can be detrimental to kidney health.

CHAPTER FIVE

Why SMOOTHIES?

Smoothies can be an excellent addition to a kidney-friendly diet. They can provide a tasty and convenient way to consume nutrient-dense foods, including fruits, vegetables, and herbs, that are beneficial for the kidneys. For example, many smoothie recipes incorporate ingredients like blueberries, kale, and spinach, which are high in antioxidants that can help protect the kidneys from damage. Additionally, certain herbs like parsley and ginger have been shown to have diuretic properties, meaning they can help promote healthy kidney function by increasing urine output and reducing fluid retention. Smoothies can also be a good source of hydration, which is essential for maintaining proper kidney function. By including kidney-friendly ingredients in smoothies, individuals can support their kidney health while enjoying a delicious and convenient snack or meal.

Smoothies are a convenient and tasty way to incorporate nutrient-dense foods into your diet. For individuals with kidney disease, it is important to consume a diet that is low in sodium, potassium, and phosphorus, while also being rich in essential vitamins and minerals. Smoothies can be a great way to achieve this balance, as they can be made with a variety of fruits, vegetables, and other kidney-friendly ingredients.

One of the primary benefits of incorporating smoothies into a kidney-friendly diet is that they can provide a rich source of antioxidants. Antioxidants are compounds that help to protect the body from damage caused by harmful molecules called free radicals. Free radicals are naturally produced by the body, but they can also be generated by external factors like pollution, radiation, and cigarette smoke. When free radicals accumulate in the body, they can damage cells and tissues, leading to inflammation and chronic diseases like kidney disease.

Fruits and vegetables are some of the richest sources of antioxidants, which is why they are often incorporated into smoothie recipes. Some of the best fruits and vegetables for kidney health include:

- Blueberries: Blueberries are high in antioxidants called anthocyanins, which have been shown to protect against oxidative stress and inflammation in the kidneys.

- Spinach: Spinach is a great source of vitamins A and C, as well as iron and calcium. It is also low in potassium and phosphorus, making it an ideal ingredient for kidney-friendly smoothies.

- Kale: Kale is another leafy green vegetable that is rich in antioxidants, as well as vitamins K, A, and C. It is also low in potassium and phosphorus, making it a good choice for individuals with kidney disease.

- Strawberries: Strawberries are high in vitamin C and fiber, and they also contain compounds called ellagic acid and flavonoids, which have been shown to have anti-inflammatory effects on the body.

- Apples: Apples are a good source of fiber and vitamin C, and they also contain a compound called quercetin, which has been shown to have antioxidant and anti-inflammatory effects.

In addition to fruits and vegetables, many other kidney-friendly ingredients can be incorporated into smoothies, such as:

- Low-fat or non-dairy milk: Low-fat or non-dairy milk can be used as a base for smoothies, providing a source of protein and calcium while also being low in potassium and phosphorus.

- Greek yogurt: Greek yogurt is high in protein and low in potassium, making it a good addition to kidney-friendly smoothies.

- Chia seeds: Chia seeds are high in fiber and omega-3 fatty acids, which have been shown to have anti-inflammatory effects on the body.

- Ginger: Ginger has anti-inflammatory and anti-nausea properties, making it a good addition to smoothies for individuals with kidney disease.

- Parsley: Parsley is a diuretic herb that can help promote healthy kidney function by increasing urine output and reducing fluid retention.

It is important to note that while smoothies can be a great addition to a kidney-friendly diet, they should be consumed in moderation. Many smoothie recipes contain high amounts of sugar, which can be detrimental to kidney health. It is also important to choose ingredients that are low in sodium, potassium, and phosphorus, as these minerals can be harmful to individuals with kidney disease when consumed in excess.

In addition to being mindful of the ingredients used in smoothies, it is also important to be aware of the portion sizes. Drinking large amounts of fluid can be taxing on the kidneys, especially for individuals with kidney disease.

Here are some additional points on the benefits of smoothies for kidney health:

- Improved hydration: One of the primary benefits of smoothies is that they can help improve hydration levels in the body. Dehydration can be harmful to the kidneys and can lead to the formation of kidney stones. By including hydrating fruits and vegetables like watermelon, cucumber, and leafy greens in your smoothies, you can increase your water intake and support optimal kidney function.

- Reduced inflammation: Chronic inflammation is a risk factor for kidney disease, and consuming a diet rich in anti-inflammatory foods can help reduce this risk. Many ingredients commonly used in smoothies, such as turmeric, ginger, and leafy greens, have potent anti-inflammatory properties that can help protect the kidneys.

- Increased nutrient intake: Smoothies can be an excellent way to increase your nutrient intake, which is important for overall health and kidney function. Many fruits and vegetables are rich in vitamins, minerals, and antioxidants that can help protect the kidneys from damage and improve their function. By blending a variety of nutrient-dense ingredients into your smoothies, you can support optimal kidney health.

- Improved digestion: Some kidney conditions, such as chronic kidney disease, can lead to digestive problems. Smoothies can be an easy-to-digest food that can help support digestive health while also providing important nutrients for the kidneys. By including ingredients like probiotic-rich yogurt or kefir, fiber-rich fruits and vegetables, and anti-inflammatory spices, you can help support optimal digestion and kidney health.

- Lowered risk of heart disease: People with kidney disease are at an increased risk of developing heart disease. Consuming a diet rich in heart-healthy nutrients can help reduce this risk. Smoothies can be an excellent way to include heart-healthy foods like berries, avocados, nuts, and seeds in your diet. These foods are rich in healthy fats, fiber, and antioxidants that can help support heart health and reduce the risk of heart disease.

In conclusion, smoothies can be a tasty and convenient way to support optimal kidney health. By including kidney-friendly ingredients like leafy greens, berries, and low-potassium fruits, and avoiding kidney-enemy foods like processed meats and high-sodium foods, you can help protect your kidneys from damage and improve their function. Additionally, by incorporating other healthy lifestyle habits like staying hydrated, reducing inflammation, and maintaining a healthy weight, you can support optimal kidney function and overall health.

CHAPTER SIX

THE BASICS OF MAKING SMOOTHIES

Making a smoothie is a straightforward process that does not require any special equipment. All you need is a blender or food processor, some fruits and vegetables, and any additional ingredients that you want to add to the smoothie.

To make a smoothie, start by selecting the fruits and vegetables you want to use. Fresh or frozen fruits and vegetables can be used, depending on your preference. You can use a single fruit or a combination of fruits to make a delicious smoothie. Some of the popular fruits used in smoothies include bananas, strawberries, blueberries, raspberries, mangoes, and pineapples. Vegetables like spinach, kale, cucumber, and carrots can also be used.

After selecting your fruits and vegetables, wash and chop them into smaller pieces to make them easier to blend. If you are using frozen fruits, allow them to thaw for a few minutes before blending.

Next, add the fruits and vegetables to the blender and add any other ingredients you want to use. You can add milk, yogurt, nut butter, honey, or any other ingredient you want to customize the taste of your smoothie. To enhance the nutritional value of your smoothie, you can add protein powder, chia seeds, flax seeds, or other superfoods.

Once all the ingredients are in the blender, blend until the mixture is smooth and creamy. Depending on the consistency you prefer, you can add more liquid or ice to your smoothie to make it thinner or thicker.

Finally, pour the smoothie into a glass and enjoy. You can also add some toppings like granola, nuts, or fresh fruit to make your smoothie more visually appealing and add texture.

Smoothies are a great way to incorporate more fruits and vegetables into your diet, and they are an easy and delicious way to take care of your kidneys. With just a few simple steps, you can make a healthy and delicious smoothie that will nourish your body and support your kidney health.

CHAPTER SEVEN

SMOOTHIES FOR PREVENTING KIDNEY HEALTH

Here are 20 smoothie recipes that can be beneficial for kidney health:

1. Blueberry Spinach Smoothie - blend blueberries, spinach, almond milk, banana, and ice

2. Pineapple Cucumber Smoothie - blend pineapple, cucumber, coconut water, lime juice, and ice

3. Strawberry Kiwi Smoothie - blend strawberries, kiwi, almond milk, banana, and ice.

4. Mango Carrot Smoothie - blend mango, carrots, orange juice, Greek yogurt, and ice

5. Green Tea Blueberry Smoothie - brew green tea, let it cool, then blend with blueberries, banana, almond milk, and ice

6. Beet Ginger Smoothie - blend cooked beets, ginger, apple juice, Greek yogurt, and ice

7. Cherry Almond Smoothie - blend cherries, almond milk, Greek yogurt, honey, and ice

8. Peach Raspberry Smoothie - blend peaches, raspberries, almond milk, honey, and ice

9. Carrot Orange Smoothie - blend carrots, orange juice, Greek yogurt, honey, and ice

10. Watermelon Mint Smoothie - blend watermelon, mint leaves, lime juice, and ice

11. Kiwi Pineapple Smoothie - blend kiwi, pineapple, coconut water, Greek yogurt, and ice

12. Kale Pineapple Smoothie - blend kale, pineapple, coconut water, Greek yogurt, and ice

13. Pomegranate Blueberry Smoothie - blend pomegranate juice, blueberries, Greek yogurt, honey, and ice

14. Spinach Avocado Smoothie - blend spinach, avocado, almond milk, banana, and ice

15. Raspberry Coconut Smoothie - blend raspberries, coconut milk, Greek yogurt, honey, and ice

16. Orange Mango Smoothie - blend oranges, mango, Greek yogurt, honey, and ice

17. Blueberry Coconut Smoothie - blend blueberries, coconut milk, Greek yogurt, honey, and ice

18. Apple Cinnamon Smoothie - blend apples, cinnamon, almond milk, Greek yogurt, and ice

19. Peanut Butter Banana Smoothie - blend peanut butter, banana, almond milk, Greek yogurt, honey, and ice

20. Turmeric Ginger Smoothie - blend turmeric, ginger, almond milk, banana, and ice.

Remember to consult with a doctor or dietitian before making any significant dietary changes, especially if you have kidney disease or any other medical conditions.

CHAPTER EIGHT

SMOOTHIES FOR MANAGING KIDNEY ISSUES

Here are 20 smoothie recipes that may help manage kidney issues or problems:

- Blueberry-Banana Smoothie: Blend 1 cup of blueberries, 1 banana, 1/2 cup of plain yogurt, and a splash of almond milk.

- Green Apple Smoothie: Blend 1 green apple, 1/2 cup of spinach, 1/2 cup of kale, 1/2 cup of plain yogurt, and a splash of water.

- Strawberry-Kiwi Smoothie: Blend 1 cup of strawberries, 1 kiwi, 1/2 cup of plain yogurt, and a splash of water.

- Peach-Mango Smoothie: Blend 1 peach, 1/2 cup of mango, 1/2 cup of plain yogurt, and a splash of almond milk.

- Pineapple-Coconut Smoothie: Blend 1 cup of pineapple, 1/2 cup of coconut milk, 1/2 cup of plain yogurt, and a splash of water.

- Cucumber-Mint Smoothie: Blend 1 cucumber, 1/4 cup of fresh mint leaves, 1/2 cup of plain yogurt, and a splash of water.

- Beet-Berry Smoothie: Blend 1 cooked beet, 1 cup of mixed berries, 1/2 cup of plain yogurt, and a splash of almond milk.

- Carrot-Orange Smoothie: Blend 1 carrot, 1 orange, 1/2 cup of plain yogurt, and a splash of water.

- Avocado-Berry Smoothie: Blend 1/2 avocado, 1 cup of mixed berries, 1/2 cup of plain yogurt, and a splash of water.

- Spinach-Berry Smoothie: Blend 1 cup of spinach, 1 cup of mixed berries, 1/2 cup of plain yogurt, and a splash of water.

- Sweet Potato-Cinnamon Smoothie: Blend 1 cooked sweet potato, 1/2 teaspoon of cinnamon, 1/2 cup of plain yogurt, and a splash of almond milk.

- Cherry-Almond Smoothie: Blend 1 cup of cherries, 1/4 cup of almonds, 1/2 cup of plain yogurt, and a splash of water.

- Raspberry-Lime Smoothie: Blend 1 cup of raspberries, juice from 1/2 lime, 1/2 cup of plain yogurt, and a splash of water.

- Blueberry-Beet Smoothie: Blend 1 cup of blueberries, 1 cooked beet, 1/2 cup of plain yogurt, and a splash of water.

- Orange-Ginger Smoothie: Blend 1 orange, 1/2 inch of fresh ginger, 1/2 cup of plain yogurt, and a splash of water.

- Banana-Nut Smoothie: Blend 1 banana, 1/4 cup of mixed nuts, 1/2 cup of plain yogurt, and a splash of almond milk.

- Cherry-Vanilla Smoothie: Blend 1 cup of cherries, 1/2 teaspoon of vanilla extract, 1/2 cup of plain yogurt, and a splash of water.

- Mango-Lime Smoothie: Blend 1/2 cup of mango, juice from 1/2 lime, 1/2 cup of plain yogurt, and a splash of water.

- Apple-Cinnamon Smoothie: Blend 1 apple, 1/2 teaspoon of cinnamon, 1/2 cup of plain yogurt, and a splash of water.

- Pineapple Cucumber Smoothie: Blend 1 cup chopped pineapple, 1/2 cup chopped cucumber, 1/2 cup water, and a handful of ice. Pineapple is rich in bromelain, an enzyme that may help reduce inflammation and promote kidney health.

- Chocolate Banana Almond Butter Smoothie: Blend 1 ripe banana, 1 tablespoon almond butter, 1 tablespoon cocoa powder, 1/2 cup almond milk, and a handful of ice. Almond butter is a good source of healthy fats and protein, which can help support kidney health.

- Apple Cinnamon Oatmeal Smoothie: Blend 1 apple, 1/4 cup rolled oats, 1/2 teaspoon cinnamon, 1/2 cup almond milk, and a handful of ice. Oats are rich in fiber and may help lower cholesterol levels, which can benefit kidney health.

- Mango Carrot Ginger Smoothie: Blend 1 cup chopped mango, 1/2 cup chopped carrots, 1 teaspoon grated ginger, 1/2 cup water, and a handful of ice. Carrots are a good source of vitamin A, which can help support kidney health.

- Blueberry Spinach Smoothie: Blend 1 cup fresh or frozen blueberries, 1 cup spinach, 1/2 cup plain Greek yogurt, 1/2 cup water, and a handful of ice. Blueberries are rich in antioxidants, which may help protect the kidneys from damage.

- Beetroot Berry Smoothie: Blend 1 small beetroot, 1/2 cup mixed berries, 1/2 cup water, and a handful of ice. Beets are rich in nitrates, which may help improve blood flow to the kidneys.

- Cherry Vanilla Smoothie: Blend 1 cup frozen cherries, 1/2 teaspoon vanilla extract, 1/2 cup plain Greek yogurt, 1/2 cup almond milk, and a handful of ice. Cherries are rich in antioxidants and may help reduce inflammation, which can benefit kidney health.

- Kale Pineapple Smoothie: Blend 1 cup chopped kale, 1 cup chopped pineapple, 1/2 cup water, and a handful of ice. Kale is a good source of vitamins A and C, which can help support kidney health.

- Strawberry Banana Chia Smoothie: Blend 1 ripe banana, 1 cup fresh or frozen strawberries, 1 tablespoon chia seeds, 1/2 cup almond milk, and a handful of ice. Chia seeds are a good source of omega-3 fatty acids, which can help reduce inflammation and support kidney health.

- Turmeric Ginger Smoothie: Blend 1 teaspoon ground turmeric, 1 teaspoon grated ginger, 1/2 cup pineapple, 1/2 cup almond milk, and a handful of ice. Turmeric and ginger are both anti-inflammatory and may help support kidney health.

CHAPTER NINE

SMOOTHIES FOR TREATING KIDNEY PROBLEMS

- Berry Blast: 1 cup mixed berries, 1 banana, 1 cup spinach, 1/2 cup unsweetened almond milk, and 1 scoop of protein powder.

- Tropical Tango: 1 cup frozen pineapple, 1/2 cup frozen mango, 1/2 cup coconut water, 1/2 cup Greek yogurt, and 1 scoop of protein powder.

- Spinach Surprise: 1 cup spinach, 1 banana, 1/2 cup unsweetened almond milk, 1/2 cup Greek yogurt, 1 tablespoon of honey, and 1 scoop of protein powder.

- Blueberry Burst: 1 cup blueberries, 1/2 cup plain kefir, 1/2 cup water, 1 tablespoon chia seeds, 1 teaspoon of honey, and 1 scoop of protein powder.

- Green Machine: 1/2 cup frozen pineapple, 1/2 cup frozen mango, 1/2 avocado, 1 cup spinach, 1/2 cup water, and 1 scoop of protein powder.

- Orange You Glad: 1 orange, 1 banana, 1/2 cup plain kefir, 1/2 cup water, 1 tablespoon of honey, and 1 scoop of protein powder.

- Banana Berry: 1 banana, 1/2 cup mixed berries, 1/2 cup plain kefir, 1/2 cup water, and 1 scoop of protein powder.

- Creamy Coconut: 1/2 cup frozen pineapple, 1/2 banana, 1/2 cup coconut milk, 1/2 cup plain Greek yogurt, 1 tablespoon of honey, and 1 scoop of protein powder.

- Almond Butter and Jelly: 1/2 cup frozen strawberries, 1/2 banana, 1/2 cup almond milk, 1 tablespoon almond butter, and 1 scoop of protein powder.

- Mango Madness: 1 cup frozen mango, 1/2 cup plain kefir, 1/2 cup water, 1 tablespoon of honey, and 1 scoop of protein powder.

- Chocolate Banana: 1 banana, 1 tablespoon cocoa powder, 1/2 cup unsweetened almond milk, 1 tablespoon honey, and 1 scoop of protein powder.

- Peach Perfect: 1 peach, 1/2 cup plain Greek yogurt, 1/2 cup water, 1 tablespoon of honey, and 1 scoop of protein powder.

- Peanut Butter Cup: 1/2 banana, 1 tablespoon peanut butter, 1/2 cup unsweetened almond milk, 1 tablespoon cocoa powder, and 1 scoop of protein powder.

- Raspberry Lemonade: 1 cup frozen raspberries, 1 lemon, juiced, 1/2 cup water, 1 tablespoon of honey, and 1 scoop of protein powder.

- Strawberry Banana: 1 banana, 1 cup frozen strawberries, 1/2 cup plain kefir, 1/2 cup water, and 1 scoop of protein powder.

- Vanilla Almond: 1/2 cup unsweetened almond milk, 1/2 cup plain Greek yogurt, 1 teaspoon vanilla extract, 1 tablespoon of honey, and 1 scoop of protein powder.

CONCLUSION

In conclusion, smoothies are a tasty and nutritious strategy for both preventing and managing kidney issues. By incorporating kidney-friendly foods and avoiding kidney-enemy foods, individuals can create a smoothie that not only tastes great but also provides important nutrients and supports kidney health. Smoothies can also be a convenient and easy way to incorporate a variety of fruits, vegetables, and other ingredients into the diet.

It is important to remember that while smoothies can be a beneficial addition to a kidney-healthy diet, they should not be relied upon as the sole treatment for kidney issues. Consulting with a healthcare professional and following their recommended treatment plan is crucial for proper kidney health management.

By understanding the basics of making smoothies, and having a variety of kidney-friendly smoothie recipes on hand, individuals can easily incorporate this delicious and nutritious beverage into their daily routine. So, raise a glass to kidney health and enjoy a delicious smoothie today!